Herbal Antibiotics

56 Little Known Natural Remedies to Help Cure and Prevent Bacterial Illnesses

Ella Marie

For more books by this author, please visit:
www.wellnessbooks.net

Table of Contents

Introduction

Bacterial infections may result from an array of sources. Yet they can prove to be very difficult to take care of. Most people reach for over-the-counter medications. When these fail to get results, they make an appointment with their doctors, and typically walk out with antibiotics to take care of the infection.

However, there are numerous herbal antibiotics that you can use at home that won't cost you a fortune. In fact, many of them you may already have available in your home. Others are easily accessible, and you can buy them online or at local retailers as well.

Herbal antibiotics don't have any side effects which is a common issue with prescription medications. On top of that, over time your body builds up a tolerance to prescription antibiotics. This can render them useless in the future if you get sick frequently.

Prescription antibiotics are also known to wreck havoc on your gut resulting in what is called dysbiosis, which is when the bad bacteria over-power the good bacteria inside your gut. This imbalance will usually result in a wide array of health issues, such as candida overgrowth and a lowering of the immune system to name a few.

Herbal antibiotics that are used to take care of bacterial infections are referred to as astringents. Adding such foods to your regular diet can boost your immune system and reduce the risk of such infections even occurring.

Herbal antibiotics can be used when you need them without any hassles or waiting periods. Most of them can be used by both children and adults. In this book, you will learn about the fifty-six different options you have!

It is also important to understand there may be times when you do need to take antibiotics prescribed by your doctor. However, when you use these natural remedies you can significantly reduce the risk of becoming ill with bacterial infections.

Chapter 1
Why Synthetic Antibiotics are a Big Problem in Today's Society

Not only do synthetic antibiotics result in harsh side effects, they are attributed to an array of issues in society today. In fact, they have been considered one of the big problems that modern medicine and science need to take a close look at.

Lack of Information

The biggest issue is most people don't even realize there are natural herbal antibiotics available that they can use. They assume their doctor knows best because that is the mindset that we have promoted in society. If the doctor says you need antibiotics, you go out and get them without asking questions.

For many people reading this book, that may be an eye-opening statement. You may even be angry that you have spent so much money for prescription antibiotics when you had other cheaper and healthier options. Yet you may not have been aware until now that they even existed or that they could help you feel better.

Unfortunately, until society as a whole is better informed that natural herbal antibiotics are a choice, the over use of synthetic antibiotics is going to continue.

Liver

The liver is a very important organ of the body. It needs to work properly in order for us to feel our very best. Using synthetic antibiotics regularly can damage the liver. This can make it harder for the body as a whole to perform the processes that keep you healthy and feeling your best.

Interact with Other Medications

If you have other health concerns, you may already be taking various prescription medications. It's possible, however, that they don't interact well with synthetic antibiotics. You may suffer more side effects, or your other medications may not work as well. This can make you vulnerable in regards to your overall well-being.

Dehydration

One of the common side effects of synthetic antibiotics is diarrhea. As a result, dehydration can occur as the body is losing fluids and electrolytes. A person may not feel thirsty, but this doesn't mean they are staying hydrated, so special care needs to be taken.

Vaginal Yeast Infections

Studies have linked the rise in vaginal yeast infections to the use of synthetic antibiotics. This is because they often kill the good bacteria as well as the harmful bacteria. The body relies on the good bacteria to keep things balanced. Even young girls can get vaginal yeast infections for this reason.

Ironically, the way most doctors treat them is to prescribe yet another antibiotic. This can become a cycle that is both uncomfortable and unhealthy. Vaginal yeast infections can cause itching, burning, and discomfort.

Creation of Superbugs due to Resistance

There are scientists and medical professionals who worry that synthetic antibiotics are creating superbugs. They are making it harder and harder to successfully treat simple bacterial infections. This is because the body will start to build up a tolerance to antibiotics. Then it becomes increasingly difficult to kill the infection with the same drugs.

This is especially a concern for young children, who tend to get sick easier and more frequently than adults. If they are given synthetic antibiotics often, they stop being as effective. This can result in a simple bacterial infection turning into something that requires hospitalization.

Hypersensitivity and Allergies

Not everyone does well with the use of synthetic antibiotics. The body can become hypersensitive or allergic to an ingredient in the medication. For example, many people are allergic to penicillin, but they aren't aware until they take it for the first time.

Their face may swell up, they may break out in a rash, or they may find breathing difficult. Such concerns require further medical attention and often additional medication to take care of the symptoms.

Cost

The cost of synthetic antibiotics continues to increase constantly. Even those with health insurance are often frustrated with co-pays and deductibles. Or they may discover that when they get to the pharmacy, their insurance doesn't cover the particular type of antibiotic that has been prescribed.

For example, amoxicillin is usually covered. Yet many patients are now resistant to its positive effects due to their body's tolerance for antibiotics. As a result, they are prescribed Z-Pac, but this is rarely covered by health insurance plans.

Risk to Children/Pets

Any time you have synthetic antibiotics in your home, there is a risk to children and pets. There is the risk they will find and consume them. An overdose of such medications can be very serious, not only for children but for adults as well.

Taking more than the daily suggested amount won't help you get better in less time. You also have to take the medication for the entire duration it was prescribed, even if you feel better. If not, there is a risk that the bacteria won't be completely destroyed and you will have to start all over again with the medication.

Huge Profits for Companies

The huge profits that pharmaceutical companies make from the sales of synthetic antibiotics amounts to billions of dollars annually. This is part of the reason why there isn't really a push to get consumers to rely on herbal antibiotics. These companies would rather make money than focus on the overall well-being of society.

Chapter 2
Often Found in Your Kitchen

Several of the natural herbal antibiotics from which you can choose are already in your kitchen. If you or your family members get bacterial infections often, add more of them to the foods you prepare. They will enhance the flavors of your foods and drinks, and offer you a natural way to remain healthy.

Apple Cider Vinegar

There are high levels of both malic and acetic acid found in apple cider vinegar. It also contains high amounts of amino acids and vitamins. It is a powerful way to fight ailments as it is antiviral, antibacterial, and anti-fungal.

Taking a spoonful in the morning and at night is a great way to fight health concerns. If you don't like the taste, you can mix it with a glass of water to dilute it.

Cabbage

The healing powers of cabbage are enormous, but too many people don't eat it. Add this to your diet at least once a week to boost your immune system. You can also drink fresh cabbage juice daily for a week to help you bounce back from a health issue that has depleted your energy.

Coconut Oil

Not only does coconut oil help reduce the risk of bacterial infections, but it can make the foods you prepare healthier. It offers plenty of overall health benefits and it also tastes great! Any recipe that calls for the use of vegetable oil can be healthier with this one simple change. You can use this several times per week as part of a healthier diet. It is small changes like this that add up the most.

Coconut oil can help to boost your immune system. It also offers anti-fungal properties and plenty of powerful antioxidants. It is believed to help improve blood sugar levels and to boost brain function. If you don't want to cook with it, add a spoonful to your coffee in the morning for a healthy boost and more energy.

Fermented Foods

What comes to mind when you think about fermented foods? Many people associate it only with alcohol. However, there are health benefits to fermented foods as they are classified as a probiotic. They will destroy harmful bacteria but not the healthy bacteria found in the body.

Some great choices in this food category include cultured vegetables and raw pickles. You can also take a daily capsule form of it that you find at the local health food store. Fermented foods offer plenty of antioxidants and necessary microorganisms. The foods offer more benefits than the capsules.

Garlic

For at least 2,000 years garlic has been used around the world as a source of medicine. It has been used for ear infections, the flu, and even the Black Plague. Garlic contains powerful antioxidants that kill harmful bacteria.

It also eliminates free radicals in the bloodstream, so the immune system becomes stronger. Allicin is the active ingredient found in garlic, and it helps with destroying both viruses and bacteria— something a prescription antibiotic isn't able to do.

Garlic can be consumed in meals in the form of cloves. It can also be made into a juice. If you don't like the taste of garlic, there are also capsules. You only need a small amount to attain the benefits; too much garlic can actually upset the stomach. If you take any type of blood thinning medication, avoid using garlic as a natural herbal antibiotic.

Ginger

Not only is ginger powerful, it has a very strong aroma. The smell is the result of the various essential oils and compounds it is comprised of. Some of these properties offer anti-inflammatory and antibacterial properties. Only a small amount of ginger should be consumed at a time.

Honey

The sweet, delicious taste of honey makes it a popular item in any kitchen. However, it also offers antibacterial properties. Many cultures relied on raw honey before synthetic antibiotics were introduced.

An antimicrobial enzyme is found in honey, and it prohibits various types of harmful bacteria from growing. It is also believed to help with the liver and to reduce toxins in the body that can destroy the immune system. Honey can be added to drinks, consumed on toast, added to hot cereal, or consumed raw.

Onion

Many people cook with onion for the flavor, but they are also helping their immune system. Onion is believed to help with treating just about anything you can imagine. This includes bacterial infections and even inflammation.

Onion contains sulfur compounds, and that is what makes it a very good herbal antibiotic. They can also help to reduce the symptoms of the common cold and the flu, which are viral—not bacterial—illnesses.

Sage

If you tend to suffer from upper respiratory infections, sage is a great option to help you feel better. Adding this to your food regularly can boost your immune system and protect against such health concerns developing. You don't need to add much sage to make a difference.

Chapter 3
Herbs

There are also plenty of herbs you may use for cooking or to create an herbal drink. There is a lengthy list of such herbs that offer you the value of natural antibiotics. You may already be using some of them.

Others you can buy locally, either fresh or dried. It is important to do your best to find high-quality herbs. The better the quality is, the more power they will be worth when fighting off bacterial infections.

Allspice

Offering exceptional antioxidants and anti-inflammatory elements, allspice is certainly something to consider for herbal antibiotics. It can be used for various recipes, so it is often a type of preventive aid. It can give the immune system a boost so you are less likely to suffer from bacterial infections and other ailments. It is quite potent and a small amount of allspice goes a long way in flavor.

Anise

This is a spice often used in Asian food dishes, but it can be added to just about anything. You don't need too much of it, though, as it does have a bold flavor. It tastes like licorice so it is often mistaken for the former in dishes.

Anise has been used as a healing herb for many centuries in Asia and around the world. Its antibacterial properties are just one of the valuable elements it offers. It also provides plenty of antioxidants.

Don't exceed a dose of 500 mg per day. If you are going to take a maximum dose, break it up into two or three doses throughout the day instead of all at once.

Basil

Add basil to most of the dishes you cook, and it will boost your immune system. Basil oil can be added to foods you don't cook, including salads. It will help you to stay healthy and if you do start to get a type of bacterial infection, it can help kill the harmful bacteria early on.

Bay Leaf

The endless benefits from bay leaf make it a popular option for those fighting bacterial infections. It also helps to reduce acne and alleviate stomach problems. The oil from bay leaf helps reduce the ability of harmful bacteria to grow. It can also fight the growth of several forms of fungi.

Cardamom

Perhaps one of the best hidden secrets relating to fighting harmful bacteria is cardamom. It contains high amounts of cineol. It is also a very common way to fight chronic bad breath.

This is a very useful herb for the treatment of sore throat and coughing. You shouldn't use cardamom if you have gall stones or if your gall bladder has been removed.

Caraway Seed

You will get the best results if you seek black caraway seed oil. For thousands of years, it has been used to help with a variety of health concerns. It is a powerful way to fight bacteria that causes deep infections that can be difficult to combat.

This oil should be taken when you feel the initial onset of such health problems. Take a teaspoon in the morning and again at night until symptoms are no longer present. If you don't like the taste, add a bit of honey to the oil. The daily recommended dose for prevention is 50 mg to 100 mg.

Chervil

The history of chervil goes very deep in many cultures around the world. It grows wild in many regions, and it didn't take long for the value to be discovered. The best way to use it is to boil some chervil leaves in a cup of apple cider vinegar. Remove the leaves and drink the concoction with a few spoons of honey mixed in to make it sweet.

Chervil is a great option to consider for a chronic cough. Such coughing can make it hard to sleep at night. Sipping on some tea made from this herb before trying to sleep can help you get the rest you really need.

Chili Peppers

There are quite a few varieties of chili peppers out there to pick from. Some have a mild heat and others have a medium or very hot heat. You don't need to consume too much of these chili peppers to reap the benefits. They can keep the body healthy and the harmful bacteria from growing.

Cinnamon

On the sweeter side of things, there is cinnamon, which also offers protection against harmful bacteria. Cinnamon can be used in baking various sweets or it can be sprinkled into drinks to make them sweeter without the use of sugar. It can help reduce the symptoms of the common cold, muscle spasms, vomiting, and inflammation.

Cloves

Not only can cloves help win the battle against bacterial infections, they can also be used to reduce pain. Placing a few boiled cloves in your mouth between the teeth and the gums can reduce pain and inflammation until you can be seen by your dentist.

Cloves can also be used to treat mild pain due to inflammation, such as the symptoms of arthritis. Cloves can help to reduce nausea and vomiting due to the flu, health concerns, or even side effects of prescription medications.

Coriander

One of the popular uses for coriander is to prevent the risk of food poisoning. It can also help fight various forms of infections that seem to be resistant to prescription antibiotics. (This resistance can happen when a person takes them too frequently). You can add it to just about any food item and it won't alter the taste.

Joint pain is often reduced with the use of coriander. Some people find it also naturally takes care of hemorrhoids for them. Women who are pregnant or nursing may use it to increase their milk flow.

Cumin

Adding a small amount of cumin to your food will enhance flavor. This is especially true of Peruvian food dishes. Cumin is a powerful antibiotic choice. It contains thymol, and this also helps improve the efficiency of prescription antibiotics, should you need to take them.

Dill

A tiny amount of dill goes a long way due to the tangy flavor it delivers to foods. Dill can also help your body fight off infections and boost your immune system. Fresh dill can be found in the summer and early part of the fall. However, you can obtain dried dill all year long. Dill has also been useful in the fight against bone loss.

It can be applied to the inside of the mouth or the throat to reduce pain. It is important not to use dill if you are taking lithium as your doctor has prescribed. Dill can result in the body not processing lithium like it should.

Fennel

Many people sprinkle fennel seeds in their food or on top of salads as a way to boost metabolism. It is a common element for effective long-term weight loss. Fennel also has anti-fungal and antibacterial properties to offer.

Lemon Balm

Not only does lemon balm taste and smell delicious, it is highly antibacterial. It is also a calming herb that has been used for centuries to help reduce stress and anxiety. It is offered as a tea, dried leaves, capsules, and extracts. Lemon balm shouldn't be used by anyone who takes thyroid medications.

Marjoram

The common cold can be debilitating, but marjoram is a good way to reduce the length of time it lingers. It offers help for both bacterial and viral ailments. It is gentle enough that many parents use it for infants and young children. Yet it is effective enough to offer help for adults, too. It is offered as an oil and dried leaves.

Marjoram is often made into a tea that can be given to children to reduce a runny nose or the effects of the common cold. It can also be used to fight a dry cough that seems to linger. Ear pain and a sore throat are also reasons to use marjoram.

Mints

Mints offer various essential oils that boost the immune system and soothe the digestive system. They may be used in various food items you buy at the store in an effort to extend shelf-life. Mints can also be added to tea in the form of oil or leaves to help reduce bacterial infections. This includes those that affect the throat and the sinuses.

Mustard

Mustard seeds can be used to make a variety of great tasting food dishes. You only need a small amount to get the value they offer. Even the smooth mustard condiment contains such seeds and has antibacterial benefits to offer.

The use of mustard can help to reduce muscle pain and inflammation. It is also a good choice for treating the common cold. Black mustard leaves can be used in salads and other food dishes. You can also take capsules to gain benefits or boil mustard seeds to make tea.

Nutmeg

There are numerous uses for nutmeg in addition to adding flavor to foods. While many people add it to sweets such as desserts, it can be added to all types of foods. It has often been used to fight E. coli and staph infections. It features antimicrobial properties that help to reduce harmful bacteria.

Nutmeg can also reduce joint pain and mouth sores. In addition, it can alleviate nausea and diarrhea. Don't use more than 120 mg per day or it can result in hallucinations.

Oregano

Oregano isn't just for enhancing the flavor of your best Italian dishes. It is also a way to remain healthy due to the great antibacterial properties it provides. The oil from oregano leaves has the most potential.

It has been compared to the value offered by the prescription antibiotic called penicillin. Some studies have indicated oregano can help kill prostate cancer cells. The use of oregano can be very good for respiratory tract issues including a cough, croup or asthma.

For such ailments, the recommended dose is 200 mg per day. It shouldn't be used by those who take medications for bleeding disorders.

Parsley

There are some definite antibiotic properties to be found in parsley. It mainly comes from the oil extracted from parsley seeds. It can fight several forms of bacteria and fungi. One of the common ailments parsley is good for is staph infection.

It can also be used to prevent and heal urinary tract infections (UTIs) and to lessen the pain from kidney stones. It can reduce the length of time the common cold lingers and reduce the risk of jaundice. It is often used for infants that suffer from colic.

Pepper

There are several types of pepper that you can use to help reduce the risk of bacterial infections or to fight them. This includes black pepper, chili pepper and cayenne. They are also useful for fighting intestinal-related issues, as well.

All pepper contains capsicum, and that is what fights bacteria. The hotter the pepper is, the more powerful it will be in fighting the bacteria. However, you need to make sure the foods you put pepper into don't become too hot for you to consume.

Rosemary

An essential oil that smells very good is rosemary. It can be used as an oil on the body or breathed in through an infuser. If you use any essential oil, you only need a few drops because they are very powerful. Don't add more than two drops of it to your bathwater.

Rosemary offers amazing benefits for the immune system. It is a type of aromatherapy that is also used for treating chronic asthma problems. It can fight against mold, fungi and bacteria.

Sage

Reducing inflammation and offsetting bacterial problems are well known benefits of sage. This is typically offered as a dried leaf that is used for cooking. However, the leaves can also be boiled and strained to make a strong tea.

Some experts believe daily intake of sage can reduce the risk of diabetes and Alzheimer's disease. It is often used to reduce the pain and pressure from a sinus infection. It can be inhaled to reduce a dry cough or swelling of the airways caused by asthma or bronchitis. The daily dose shouldn't exceed 2.5 mg.

Tarragon

Initially, tarragon was a natural antibiotic used to prevent food poisoning in various dishes. It was considered a great preservative that allowed food to have a longer shelf-life and without consumers becoming ill. Tarragon was also an early medicine for intestinal concerns and to fight tuberculosis.

It can also be a natural way to promote better sleep habits. Too often, a person will feel groggy when they take over-the-counter or prescription sleep aids. Tarragon can help you to sleep well without that difficult side effect to contend with.

The dose to take depends on one's age and the severity of the ailment. It is best to start out with just a small amount and see how it works for you. Slowly increase the dose if you need to in order to get the most benefits.

Thyme

Another option for cooking and reducing bacterial problems is thyme. It is typically used for chronic dry coughing. It is also a good resource for those that suffer from breathing problems including asthma and bronchitis. Thyme can help to soothe the digestive tract as well.

Thyme can help with whooping cough, even when it is affecting young children. It can treat laryngitis and sore throat. If the tonsils are swollen, it can help with reducing the pain and inflammation.

Turmeric

A natural spice often found in dishes from the Middle East is turmeric. The main ingredients offer the ability to block enzymes that allow harmful bacteria to spread. Turmeric has properties that help reduce bacterial infections, inflammation, and various forms of chronic infections. It can also assist with chronic headaches and bronchitis.

Even though turmeric is spicy, it can be a natural cure for heartburn. For those that love spicy foods but not the after-effects, this can be a dream come true! It can also reduce pain and inflammation from mild to moderate arthritis.

Chapter 4
Extracts

Perhaps you have heard about the value of various extracts. These are often capsules that contain ingredients that have been created to benefit your overall health and well-being. If you already use one of these daily extracts as a supplement, you are fighting off bacterial infections without even realizing it!

These extracts aren't expensive and they can make a significant change in the way you feel. Consider what these extracts offer so you can pick one that best fits your needs.

Colloidal Silver

Various properties offered by colloidal silver include killing bacteria and germs. This extract, which is actually a mineral, has been used for more than 100 years to kill bacteria and fungi. It has also been used to take care of an array of viruses.

Colloidal silver can also help with the healing process of topical wounds and open sores that don't seem to heal as they should. It can be very helpful for those suffering from bronchitis. It can also increase energy in those suffering from chronic fatigue.

This mineral should only be used in small amounts. Make sure you follow the usage instructions on the supplement packaging. The potency of colloidal silver can vary from one product to the next.

Chrysanthemum Lavandulifolium Extract

This particular extract has a very similar makeup to that of synthetic antibiotics. It is believed to be one of the oldest products used by various cultures to cure health concerns. It can also help to boost the immune system by promoting the replication of the healthy cells.

Echinacea

The recovery time from a bacterial infection or fungal infection can be reduced with the use of echinacea. It can help with lessening the symptoms and duration of ear infections, respiratory infections and sinus problems. It also reduces inflammation, so a sore throat won't be as debilitating.

Most people take echinacea as a capsule supplement. If the oil is used, a few drops should be taken from a dropper in a glass of water once per day. Many people like to make echinacea tea with a small amount of honey to sweeten the taste.

Grapefruit Seed Extract

The vibrant antioxidants found in grapefruit are commonly known. Yet not everyone is a fan of the taste of the fresh fruit or juice. Others choose to sweeten it with a lot of sugar, but that can cause other health problems down the road.

A positive solution is the consumption of grapefruit seed extract. It offers anti-fungal and antibacterial elements. Studies have found more than 800 types of bacteria and more than 100 types of bacteria can be killed by this extract. The good news, too, is that it won't kill the healthy bacteria your body needs.

Lavender Oil

Many people rely on lavender oil to help them relax and sleep better. This essential oil is also well known for reducing inflammation. It is also an antibacterial extract that can reduce respiratory problems, sinus infections and bacterial infections that affect the throat and the ears.

Lavender oil can reduce infections all over the body in terms of severity and duration. You only need a few drops of lavender oil as it is very potent. You can add the drops to your bath water or you can put them into a diffuser.

Neem Oil

A small amount of neem oil goes a long way for overall health benefits. This oil comes from the neem tree. The leaves are also available to purchase, but the oil has the most value for your body. Neem has been used for more than 4,000 years in India and Africa to help improve skin and reduce the amount of time it takes for the body to heal.

Neem oil also helps to reduce the growth of both viruses and bacteria. At the same time, it is a natural pain reliever and it can help to reduce inflammation. It can bring down a high fever in a short amount of time. Often, it is used to reduce the effects of nausea and an upset stomach, which can be side effects of various prescription medications.

Pau d'Arco

Some people assume pau d'arco comes from France due to its name, but it is actually native of South America. The main ingredient in this herb is lapachol, which can reduce infections caused by bacteria, fungus, and viruses. Some experts also believe it has properties that can help fight certain forms of cancer.

However, most people use it as relief from the common cold. There are those that will tell you that if they take pau d'arco as soon as they feel the early symptoms of a cold, they are fine within a few days. They don't feel the severity of the cold, and it doesn't linger.

Others decide to use a low dose of pau d'arco daily during the cold and flu season. They do so as a way to boost the immune system and reduce the risk of becoming ill. This is especially true of those that work around lots of other people, as they tend to be more vulnerable to such airborne ailments.

Seed Nut Extract

While seed nut extract is often used to control diabetes, it also has plenty of antioxidants to offer. It can be used to control problems with glycemic index (GI) and chronic bacterial infections.

You can purchase seed nut as a capsule to be taken daily as prevention. However, the best benefits come from the oil that is extracted from the seed nut. This essential oil is powerful, so you only need a few drops at a time.

Tea Tree Oil

Tea tree oil was used by medical professionals until the 1940s when they started using penicillin, yet it is still considered one of the best natural antibiotics available. It comes from the leaf of the plant which is native to New South Wales and Australia. It is both antibacterial and antiviral. It is powerful enough to treat MRSA and other staff infections.

This essential oil is very powerful and should be used conservatively. Only a drop or two is necessary to get results. You can use the leaves and boil them, but the best results come from the extracted oil version.

Chapter 5
From Plants

Quite a few natural herbal antibiotics come from plants. They were used by ancient cultures to help prevent illness and cure various ailments. They can also help you to stay healthy or fight a bacterial infection.

Aloe Vera

The plant known as aloe vera is one most people have used for soothing burns. This includes cooking burns and sunburns. This plant grows in climates that are hot and dry. It can also help to fight bacterial infections and even herpes.

To use aloe, just cut open the leaves of a plant and get the sap from it. You can boil it and breathe in the vapors to help the body to recover from health ailments. For burns, it is applied directly to the affected area. Some people create aloe juice and drink it to boost their immune system.

There are also capsule supplements of aloe vera available that can be used for an array of health concerns. The daily recommended dose is between 100 mg and 200 mg per day.

Cryptolepis

This is a flowering plant that is native to Gambia and Congo. Cryptolepis is extracted from the root of the plant. It is often used as a means of treating malaria and type II diabetes. The antibacterial elements make this a very potent entity in the fight against inflammation and harmful bacteria.

Cryptolepis can be found in a variety of forms. The powder and the capsules are very common. The tea offers more benefits for the body but the taste can be bitter. Adding some honey or nectar can make the taste more enjoyable.

Echinacea

For hundreds of years, echinacea has been used to give the immune system some help. It has also been used to fight infections of both the bacterial and viral variety. This is a very potent herb, and it can destroy serious forms of bacteria, including those that cause staph infections and MRSA.

Echinacea seems to be one of the popular, go-to, herbal antibiotics. This is because it helps with such a wide range of health concerns. It can be taken daily in low doses to help prevent bacterial and viral problems. It can also be reached for quickly when you sense an illness coming on.

Many people find that echinacea helps them naturally feel better. There are very few people out there that don't get a positive response health-wise when they use it. There are both capsules and liquid forms offered at most health food stores.

Eucalyptus

The oil that comes from eucalyptus has been used around the world for thousands of years. It is native to Australia and it has been used as a pharmaceutical antiseptic. To extract the oil, the leaves are boiled or steamed.

The extraction process can be difficult and time consuming. That is why it is so expensive. Eucalyptus oil should never be applied directly to the skin without being diluted. If you do so, it can result in burning and itching of the skin. The negative effects can counter the positive ones, so always make sure you dilute it. This oil should never be taken by mouth.

This is a great option for someone who hasn't had success with other herbal antibiotics or even much relief from synthetic antibiotics. Such health concerns can include chronic sinus infections and chronic ear infections.

Juniper

The juniper plant is well known for the great tasting berries it offers. They are found in various foods and beverages to add flavor. This is an antibiotic form of herbal medicine that is often overlooked. It can help reduce problems due to bronchitis or inflammation. It can also fight bacterial infections.

For health benefits, juniper oil is a good choice. The dose is about 100 mg per day. If you use actual berries, the dose is only 1o g per day. It can be hard to get fresh juniper berries all year long, but the oil can be found online or from a health food store.

Licorice

The great smell and taste of licorice makes it enticing for both children and adults. It offers antibacterial and anti-fungal properties. It is often used to reduce inflammation. It is a good choice for chronic problems with bronchitis and viral infections.

Licorice helps the immune system so it can be used to fight off the common cold and the flu. It is best used in small amounts though. The whole root offers the best medicinal value. It shouldn't be used by anyone with high blood pressure.

If you have a sore throat or strep throat, creating a tea made from honey and licorice root can sooth it quickly. Add 1 teaspoon of licorice powder to 8 ounces of hot water. Drink twice a day until you feel better.

Olive Leaf

There is no denying the overall benefits from olive leaf. These include reducing inflammation, eliminating harmful bacteria, and strengthening the immune system. It is often used by those who suffer from arthritis and digestive problems.

The daily recommended dose to treat ongoing health concerns is 30 mL. For prevention, the dose is between 10 mL and 20 mL per day. It can be taken by mouth in the liquid form, but you shouldn't exceed 2 tablespoons per day.

Chapter 6
From Trees

A few options for herbal antibiotics come from trees. While this list is shorter and lesser known, it doesn't make of them lesser or unaccessible options.

Goldenseal Root

While goldenseal root isn't as widely known as other herbal antibiotics, it shouldn't be overlooked. It can win the battle over fungus and bacteria. It is also used to reduce chronic inflammation. This is a very potent plant and it can reduce swelling in the throat quickly.

It soothes the lining of the mucous membranes, which can become irritated by respiratory problems or a sinus infection. Goldenseal root can also reduce a chronic dry cough that inhibits sleep.

Poke Root

Poke root is very strange-looking, and it grows in the rich soil areas of North America. This root can be very useful for fighting bacteria and giving the immune system some help. You do have to be careful using it, however, as too much poke root can be poisonous. Don't use more than one drop per day or it can cause damage to the kidneys.

Usnea

Mostly known as an antioxidant, usnea is also a great way to fight harmful bacteria. It can also keep forms of fungus at bay and help you maintain a very healthy immune system. This is a great option for someone dealing with a chronic cough. Usnea soothes the mucus membranes.

Woodworm

While woodworm is mainly used to treat infections of worms, it can also help with Crohn's disease and inflammation problems. It is an herbal antibiotic that helps the body to fight off bacterial and viral problems.

Woodworm is an essential oil that should be used in small amounts. It can be found as a capsule as well. Don't exceed 5 g of this substance daily.

Chapter 7
Best Herbal Choices for Various Ailments

Selecting the best herbal antibiotics for various ailments is important. While most of them have the means to kill harmful bacteria, others also take care of harmful fungus and viruses. There are also those that boost your immune system.

Each person will react to herbal antibiotics differently. This is because each individual's body chemistry is different. You may need to experiment with a few options before you find what helps you to get well or to use as prevention.

What you choose to use may also vary based on the health concerns you are immediately facing. When you don't feel well, you need a quick solution to help you return to feeling your very best in the least amount of time.

In order to successfully fight bacterial and viral health problems, you should do all you can in order to feel your best. It's important to realize the potential of herbal options. Here is a quick reference list that you will find beneficial.

- Acne — aloe vera, calendula, tea tree oil
- Alcohol use — kudzu, primrose
- Allergies — chamomile
- Alzheimer's disease — ginkgo bilbao, rosemary
- Angina — hawthorn, garlic, green tea, willow
- Anxiety — chamomile, hops, kava, lavender, passion flower, valerian

- Arthritis — capsicum, ginger, turmeric
- Athlete's Foot — tea tree oil
- Bronchitis — echinacea
- Burns — aloe vera
- Common cold — andrographis, echinacea, licorice root
- Cough — eucalyptus
- Depression — St. John's wort
- Diarrhea — bilberry, raspberry
- Dizziness — gingko, ginger
- Earache — echinacea
- Eczema — chamomile
- Flu — echinacea
- Gingivitis — green tea, goldenseal
- Hay fever — butter bur
- High blood pressure — garlic, hawthorn
- High cholesterol — apple, cinnamon, flaxseed
- Hot flashes — red clover, soy
- Indigestion — chamomile, ginger, peppermint
- Infection — echinacea, garlic, ginseng, tea tree oil
- Insomnia — hops, kava, valerian
- Lower back pain — caracole, thymol, willow bark
- Migraines — butterbur, feverfew
- Morning sickness — ginger
- Muscle pain — capsicum, wintergreen
- Nausea — ginger
- Sore throat — licorice, mullein
- Stuffy nose — echinacea
- Toothache — clove oil, willow
- Yeast infection — garlic, goldenseal, pau d'arco

Chapter 8
Talking to your Doctor about Herbal Antibiotics

Don't be shy if you would like to talk to your doctor about herbal antibiotics. Armed with the information you have learned here, you may want to try using some of these remedies instead of synthetic antibiotics.

You should have a good enough relationship with your doctor that you can communicate with him or her openly. Let him or her know why you are going to try herbal antibiotics. Keep in mind that there may be times when you or someone in your family does need a prescription.

However, you can let your doctor know you are going to try natural antibiotics both as prevention and treatment. If you aren't able to take care of the bacteria that is causing problems, return to the doctor for an assessment and try synthetic antibiotics at that time if deemed necessary.

Most medical professionals are going to respect your decision. They can put notes in your medical files as well as in the files for your children. They will appreciate your honesty, and they will ask you to report to them if you have any questions or concerns.

Many medical professionals support the use of herbal antibiotics. However, they aren't able to promote them to their patients due to their type of business. If you have a doctor that tries to convince you not to use herbal antibiotics, you may want to reconsider your choice of who you turn to for medical care.

Even if they don't agree with your choice, most professionals are going to respect the decisions you have made. It is very important for you and your doctor to be on the same page regarding your healthcare needs and the needs of your family. Don't hide the fact that you use herbal antibiotics from your doctor.

Chapter 9
Tips for Getting the Best Possible Herbal Antibiotics

It is extremely important to understand that the quality of natural herbal antibiotics influences their value and effectiveness. It makes sense to ensure you get the best possible options. Don't cut corners with cost only to end up with a product that doesn't work like it should.

Research Before You Buy

Don't assume one product is the same as all of the rest. Be a well-informed consumer. Do your research before you buy any herbal antibiotics. Take the time to read online reviews to see what people have to say.

Read the ingredients as well, because you will be amazed at what is sometimes added that you don't want. Pay attention to online reviews from real consumers. They are far more valuable than testimonials you find about products. Consumer reviews tell you what they bought, what they used the product for, and the results they received.

While herbal antibiotics work differently for people based on their body chemistry, you can get a good idea of what may work for you. If it seems to work well for the majority of uses, it is a good product to consider trying.

Credible Online Sites

You may be able to get some amazing deals on herbal antibiotics when you buy them online. However, you do need to make sure you buy them from a credible online site.

Find out how long the business has been open. Remember, anyone can create a professional-looking website. You need to find out how long they have been selling and how many complaints they have received.

Will you get a tracking number when your order ships? What is the quality of their customer support? Is there any type of refund policy or guarantee offered?

Take the time to compare several websites so you can get a realistic idea of what is offered. Make sure you compare the pricing and the shipping, too. Sometimes, you will find a lower price but when you add on the shipping it causes a huge jump in overall cost.

If there is a place to enter a promo code or discount code, open up a second browser and search for one. By copying and pasting what you find, you will save money each time you order.

Buy Fresh Herbs When Possible

If you plan to use herbs you can cook with your herbal antibiotics, try to buy them fresh. You may be able to get them at the produce department of your grocery store. Depending on the time of year, there may be farm markets around you that offer them.

Remember, adding such fresh herbs to the foods you cook can be a great line of defense from bacterial and viral health concerns. These herbs can also enhance the taste of the food you serve for your family.

Grow Your Own Herbs

There are also kits you can buy that help you to grow your own herbs. This is less expensive than buying fresh ones locally. You don't need a large amount of space to grow them. In fact, some of these kits are small enough that you place them on the windowsill in your kitchen.

Follow Dosage Instructions Completely

Never exceed the dosing instructions for herbal antibiotic products. Too often, people will increase the dose thinking it will help them to get better in less time. That isn't true though and it can result in side effects or serious illness.

When the dosage has low and high options, start out with the lowest possible dose. If you don't feel you are getting the maximum benefit, then you can gradually increase your intake until you reach the appropriate threshold. If the directions say to divide the product up into two or three doses per day, don't take it all at once.

Proper Storage

Don't overlook properly storing herbal antibiotics. Generally, you need to keep them away from light, heat, and moisture. Don't store supplements in the bathroom due to the moisture caused by showering. Don't place any medications or herbal products on a counter where they can be exposed to sunlight.

Instead, store them in a cool, dark location that is also dry. Keep a good eye on expiration dates, too. Make sure you keep all herbal products and other forms of medications out of the reach of children or pets.

Using Essential Oils

The potency of essential oils is important to understand. A few drops diluted in water can be more than significant. Most essential oils shouldn't be applied directly to the skin without diluting them. They shouldn't be consumed orally either.

Never mix essential oils together unless you are following a specific recipe. Otherwise, you could create some adverse reactions that aren't appealing and won't help you accomplish your health goals.

Conclusion

Bacterial infections can be hard to avoid due to the constant exposure we have to germs and to other people. However, their symptoms can be severe and can keep energy levels and quality of life low. A bacterial infection rarely gets better on its own, and it can deplete your immune system in no time at all.

Prescription antibiotics are often very expensive, even if you have insurance coverage. They can also create an array of side effects, such as nausea, diarrhea, dry mouth, insomnia and shaking. None of those side effects are easy to deal with.

The use of natural herbal antibiotics has been taking place since the beginning of time. In many cultures, there were people who would go out and collect the herbs and extracts. They would offer these items to those that were suffering from symptoms of bacterial infections.

You are now aware of fifty-six possible options for naturally preventing and curing bacterial infections. You may have to experiment with some of the options to find what works best for you! Do your part to stay as healthy as possible.

This includes getting at least eight hours of sleep each night and daily exercise. Eat a well-balanced diet with minimum amounts of sugar. Practice relaxation techniques including meditation and communication to reduce stress. Maintain healthy relationships and avoid dangerous lifestyle habits including drinking and smoking.

Keeping your body healthy is going to help you attain the quality of life you want. The use of natural herbal antibiotics can help boost your immune system and bounce back if you should be affected by a bacterial infection.

Studies over the past several decades indicate frequent use of antibiotics result in antibiotic-resistant infections. This means a simple illness could result in hospitalization or even death because the body isn't able to use those antibiotics successfully to get well.

Did you Like "Herbal Antibiotics"?

Before you go, I'd like to say thank you so much for purchasing my book.

I know you could have picked from dozens of books on this subject, but you took a chance with mine, and I'm truly grateful for that.

So, once again, a big thanks for downloading this book and reading all the way to the end—I truly appreciate it.

Now I'd like to ask for a small favor if you don't mind:

Would you be so kind as to take a minute of your time and leave a review for this book on Amazon?

This feedback will help me continue to write the kind of books that help you get results. And if you loved it, then please feel free to let me know! :)

More Books By Ella Marie:

Baking Soda Cure: Discover the Amazing Power and Health Benefits of Baking Soda, its History and Uses For Cooking, Cleaning, and Curing Ailments

Essential Oils For Beginners: The Little Known Secrets to Essential Oils and Aromatherapy for Weight Loss, Beauty and Healing

Yoga For Beginners: The Ultimate Beginner Yoga Guide to Lose Weight, Relieve Stress and Tone Your Body With Yoga

Leptin Resistance: The Ultimate Leptin Resistance Diet Guide For Weight Loss Including Delicious Recipes And How to Overcome Leptin Resistance Naturally

DASH Diet For Weight Loss: The Ultimate Beginner Dash Diet Guide For Weight Loss, Lower Blood Pressure, and Better Health Including Delicious Dash Diet Recipes

Mindfulness For Beginners: 25 Easy Mindfulness Exercises To Help You Live In The Present Moment, Conquer Anxiety And Stress, And Have A Fulfilling Life with Mindfulness Meditation

Vegan Slow Cooker: The Ultimate Vegan Slow Cooker Cookbook Including 39 Easy & Delicious Vegan Slow Cooker Recipes For Breakfast, Lunch & Dinner!